The Anti-Inflammatory Diet

Thank You Gift

I want to say Thank You for buying my book so I put together a thank you gift especially for readers.

This page contains a quick reference guide to gluten, fats and oils is for you to print off and keep handy in the kitchen so visit the link below to get access.

www.BlueBeanPublishing.com/Anti-Inflammatory

Table of Contents

The Anti-Inflammatory Diet

Heath Easton

INTRODUCTION

Inflammation: The word is everywhere these days.

In newspaper headlines, thrown around online in blogs and articles; the inflammation word pops up everywhere and anywhere health is discussed.

The problem is, not everyone is clear on what inflammation is or why it matters. So, **what** is inflammation and **why** does it matter to you?

Inflammation is a natural and healthy response to injury or damage (not just physical damage – diet, stress and other lifestyle factors can all cause damage), which the body uses to kick-start the healing process. This is **acute** inflammation – the **essential and normal reaction** to isolated incidents of damage – getting a cut, eating something you're allergic to, a sunburn etc.

That sounds ok… so what's the issue?

The problem is in our marvelous, modern-day lives, there are often factors that **cause low levels of prolonged inflammation** in our bodies. Inflammation is supposed to be short and sweet, but when the inflammatory process doesn't shut down it becomes constant and throws the body into imbalance, which causes a host of problems. Poor diet, lack of sleep, stress, and improper exercise can all contribute towards this **chronic inflammation**, which can be hugely problematic.

This level of inflammation has been linked to an array of health issues, including **obesity, diabetes, heart disease, arthritis, and depression** among others.

So, does inflammation affect **you** and is there anything you can **do** about it?

Absolutely – this is where I'm here to help!

By learning a little bit about **what inflammation is, what causes it** and **how to fight it,** you'll be able massively **improve your health** using a few small diet and lifestyle changes.

Inside you'll learn:
• Exactly how inflammation works in both an acute and chronic way

- Signs you may be suffering from chronic inflammation
- What factors cause inflammation – lifestyle issues, diet, exercise among other

- Powerful tools for fighting inflammation in your body

- The anti-inflammatory diet, including my favorite anti-inflammatory recipes

- Top tips and strategies for reducing inflammation and becoming healthier

PART 1:

UNDERSTANDING

INFLAMMATION

INFLAMMATION IN THE MODERN ENVIRONMENT

You may not often consider that although your body is hurting, it is also trying to heal you, but that is often the case in the modern environment. Chronic and certain types of acute inflammation are either direct causes of deadly diseases or they are detrimental, deteriorating, side effects of many bodily processes. We have all seen inflammation in the form of a twisted ankle or a scrape and we have seen it heal completely or form a protective scar. What we don't often see is that internal inflammation can be chronic or acute and can cause long-term damage along with a whole range of side effects that can make daily life painful and difficult.

What is Inflammation?

Inflammation is pretty easy to recognize when it is near the skin. There are several signs of inflammation, most easily recognized when it is acute, as in when you scrape your knee or jam your finger. The signs are heat, redness, swelling, immobility and pain. To varying degrees, these same signs and symptoms will be present during chronic and internal inflammation and are important factors which initially promote healing.

Inflammation is part of the innate immune response; this means that it heals and protects the body, but unlike the immune response that targets specific bacteria, inflammation is a generic first response to changes in the body and has several different triggers. These triggers can be set off by physical damage, but inflammation can be triggered by many other factors like stress and diet. The role of inflammation is damage control, forming a protective barrier, limiting further damage and starting the repair process. It not only assists in preventing infection, but also removes damaged and dying tissue. The problem with inflammation is that it is a type of panic response by your body and if it becomes prolonged or constant, can cause collateral damage and possibly lead to a cycle of chronic damage and attempted healing.

Stages of Inflammation

Inflammation is a response to damage or irritation, but it can also be a response to something your body perceives as a threat. Inflammation also responds to infections because they can cause damage, but also gain entry through open wounds. The first step of inflammation is your body recognizing damage or recognizing a potential threat to the body. Certain chemical and hormone reactions, usually stress or toxic diets, can also trigger inflammation when there is no damage. Once the damage is recognized, mast cells and basophils release the chemical histamine. Most of us recognize histamines as the chemical that makes us itch, but it does a lot more. In the bloodstream, histamine dilates the blood vessels enough to allow the first responder cells to get out through now open gaps in the vessel wall and get to the damaged area. The gaps in the vessel can allow a lot of fluid out and this is what causes swelling, which can be minor or can cause a softball sized ankle. The rush of blood causes both the redness and the heat, which are common symptoms of inflammation.

As the vessels are dilating, mast cells, which are located within various tissues and not in the blood, release a variety of chemicals. Mast cells are vitally important as a first step to recognizing pathogens entering the body and can release messenger cells to alert the body to send the right antibodies. Another primary function is to release prostaglandins, which bind to nerves and cause pain and can even work to cause a fever. While pain and fever seem like completely negative side effects, they exist for good reasons.

Pain is purposely inflicted by inflammation to give a warning to your brain to try not to use that part of your body. If you didn't have pain, you would be less likely to rest that part of your body and could cause further injury. So, while the pain is bad, it does serve as a useful reminder not to walk on that sprained ankle or poke that cut or bruise. When inflammation goes overboard, then that pain can be quite an inconvenience. No one likes a fever and it can be dangerous, but it is also important because it can create too hostile of an environment for invading pathogens to survive. In ideal cases, fever helps kill off invaders and as soon as the invaders are gone, the fever breaks, leading you to feel better fast. However, chronic or unregulated inflammation caused by lack of sleep, stress or poor diet, can lead to low level fevers that can make you feel hot, weak and tired.

So, now that your wound hurts and you know not to use it, your body goes to work attacking any invading pathogens, foreign bodies or dead or misplaced bodily cells. There are an amazing variety of cells that work together to respond to injury. Some cells surround individual bacteria and allow them to be safely eaten by white blood cells known as macrophages. These macrophages also respond to foreign objects such as a splinter and can join together to create a barrier between the invader and the rest of the body. After dealing with the trauma, the body gets to work trying to repair itself, which is quite a feat as there is a large amount of fluid, dead cells and bacteria and healthy tissue is often damaged in the crossfire as well.

In an ideal situation the inflammatory process is able to shut down after the pathogens have been dealt with. The best outcome is a perfect response to damage resulting in cells cleaning up the debris and healing back to the body's natural state. This is often the case with a small cut and a rolled ankle. Healing can also be difficult if there is a large amount of tissue destruction and the body can't regenerate the tissues and simply covers the wound with a collagen material. This results in the smooth lasting scars and while they are not as functional as normal skin, they are protective and allow skin and even ligaments and tendons to function to some degree. If the body cannot handle the invading object or pathogen, it can wall it off from the rest of the body and form an abscess. Where inflammation becomes a major problem is when it can't shut off in the ways described above and becomes persistent and prolonged.

CHRONIC INFLAMMATION

While acute inflammation can be painful and ugly bruises can last for days, after it is resolved, your body can usually go back to working the way it used to. **With chronic inflammation, your body is continuously in panic mode**, trying to fix something or being forced to respond to low-level traumas. While acute inflammation can cause short term damage, that damage is often healed by the same inflammatory response; chronic inflammation causes repeated damage which can create a build-up of scar tissue, disfigure and erode joints, and can cause wounds to remain unhealed indefinitely. Chronic inflammation can eventually cause serious damage that may affect multiple organs from the heart to the kidneys to the digestive tract.

The previously mentioned macrophages, the large white blood cells that consume bacteria and other fragments, as well as other immune cells release reactive oxygen species, which are oxygen containing chemicals. Reactive oxygen is deadly to invading pathogens and various chemicals, including hydrogen peroxide are carried by immune cells such as macrophages and used to neutralize pathogens. **The bad news is that these chemicals, once released, also damage other body tissues and cause oxidative damage**. Oxidants damage the DNA of a cell and can cause a variety of problems including premature ageing and they can cause cancer. At the site of inflammation however, the reactive oxygen species cause continued damage, which only continues a cycle of inflammation.

Chronic Inflammatory Disorders

Chronic inflammation can cause or worsen a wide variety of serious health conditions, such as **obesity, heart disease, arthritis to depression, and acne**. But poor diet can lead to poor gut health and increased intestinal permeability, which in itself, is associated with a number of inflammatory conditions like **celiac disease, inflammatory bowel disease, irritable bowel syndrome, food allergies, eczema and psoriasis**. Links are even appearing between gut health and mental conditions like **autism and schizophrenia.**

Inflammatory Triggers

So how does chronic inflammation occur? Inflammation is

a complex process as it involves dozens of specific cells and multiple chemicals and there are many ways the process can go wrong and many ways it can be repetitively triggered. We'll dig into these in more detail in the next chapter, but some of the causes of inflammation are:

- Toxic diets
- Poor gut health
- Lack of sleep
- Chronic stress
- Lack of movement
- Insufficient recovery from exercise
- Lack of relaxation time

Diet and Inflammation

One of the biggest factors that will influence inflammation is your daily diet. You are a product of what you eat and even if you suffer from one of the other inflammatory triggers mentioned below, your diet can have a profound effect, either worsening or improving the symptoms. Diet creates a double whammy on inflammation as **foods themselves can promote inflammation and also compromise gut health, leading to further inflammation**. The most detrimental aspects of the modern western diet are the abundance of refined sugars, processed foods, gluten and industrial fats.

Spikes in blood glucose promote inflammation in the body. Although the mechanism of action is still under investigation, one way this happens is through the depression of antioxidants in the bloodstream following a spike in blood glucose[1]. Excess sugar and carbohydrates also cause obesity and insulin resistance, which also have an inflammatory effect. Our modern diet, however, is flooded with excess sugar - any meal can contain far more sugar than our bodies are able to handle at once and we often eat far more sugar than we should. This constant elevating of blood sugar is literally toxic to the body and it is quite possible to sustain dangerous blood sugar levels, even without being diabetic.

Like sugar, fats also have a large impact on inflammation. Omega-3 fatty acids help to form anti-inflammatory eicosanoids, which work to signal the inflammatory response to slow or stop inflammation and help it from having a runaway reaction. Omega-6 acids on the other hand, form the production of inflammatory versions of eicosanoids and **improper balance of omega-3 to omega-6 can lead to an inflammatory reaction,** with less of an ability to stop it.

Trans fats (industrially hydrogenated oils like margarine) are particularly bad as they promote a bad balance of HDL and LDL cholesterol, which leaves plaque in the arteries that the body treats as an invader and attacks with inflammation. Trans fat also interacts with the cells forming the walls of blood vessels and can interfere with how they open and close to start and stop the rush of fluid of an inflammatory response. The wrong balance of the wrong fats can cause inflammation to go haywire, while a balance of fats can go a long way towards regulating inflammation.

Aside from these basic components, there are many chemicals used in food that are triggers for inflammation. **Two of the biggest culprits that may be wreaking havoc on your body are dairy and wheat products.** Lactose intolerance is one of the most common food allergies and the inflammatory impact of gluten is now becoming more understood. It is clear that many people aren't equipped to drink milk past infancy and we have eaten wheat for a very short time in relation to our evolutionary history.

Although bread is major part of many people's diets and many health authorities promote whole grain consumption, it contains potent anti-nutrients that can have an anti-inflammatory effect on the body.
Gliadin (a component of gluten) and wheat germ agglutinin (WGA) found in wheat (our biggest source of gluten) are known to compromise the integrity of the gut and promote an immune response, leading to – you guessed it – inflammation[2].

For some, reactions may be severe enough for them to avoid dairy or wheat; however, these foods can still cause inflammation throughout the digestive system and beyond without showing any symptoms. Over half of the population has a sensitivity or difficulty digesting either dairy or wheat, but many have no idea.

Aside from these two bigger inflammatory foods, there are many other products that produce inflammation. Excessive alcohol consumption causes inflammation of the mouth, oesophagus, and stomach, in addition to the many other problems it can cause. Food additives like MSG and artificial sweeteners have complex inflammatory effects that are still being studied and many people can be sensitive to any number of the hundreds of chemicals which can go into modern processed foods. Finally, probiotic bacteria can help regulate inflammation as these bacteria form an important part of the immune system. Many things influence the proper balance of gut bacteria and an unbalanced system caused by high carb diets or abuse of antibiotics or many other factors can lead to improper immune response that can take a long time to resolve.

Anti-Inflammatory Foods

Just as inflammation can be incredibly complex, reducing inflammation is also complex. Medications such as steroids will reduce inflammation, but they also suppress the immune system and can have a variety of side-effects. Fortunately, there are multiple foods that reduce inflammation in a variety of different ways and can easily be enjoyed in moderation. Many problems caused by inflammation stem from the fact that the body is stuck in an endless inflammatory cascade and attempted healing is impeded by collateral inflammation damage. If the cause of inflammation was removed and the inflammatory response was able to be controlled, then the body could start to heal. It is not unusual for many inflammatory disorders to be completely managed or cured simply by changing to an anti-inflammatory diet, though following the lifestyle tips in the following section will help too. Removing inflammatory foods and finding a way to incorporate anti-inflammatory foods can drastically improve your health and will help regulate and remove inflammation you may not have realized you had. The good thing is that there is no shortage of food that can help regulate inflammation.

Foods to Include

(See the next section for more info)

A diet rich in whole, unprocessed, natural foods will be innately rich in anti-inflammatory ingredients – a variety of different colored vegetables & fruit, meat, fish, nuts & seeds, natural oils & fats and herbs & spices. Detoxifying and anti-oxidant foods such as leafy green vegetables, beets and some spices can help limit and reverse many of the effects of inflammation while removing toxins in the body that can trigger inflammation. Oily fish can provide anti-inflammatory omega-3 and certain oils such as olive oils and those found within nuts help to balance your body's good and bad fats and cholesterol. Foods high in natural fiber like fruits and vegetables go well like probiotic foods such as kombucha, kefir or the standard yogurt which helps to regulate the millions of good bacteria in your digestive system.

Finally, there are multiple foods that reduce the body's inflammatory response through the specific compounds they contain, some of which are still not fully understood. Spices such as cinnamon, turmeric and ginger are some of the most potent dietary anti-inflammatories and can sometimes be as effective as specific anti-inflammatory medicines. Green tea, as well as many other types of tea such as lemongrass, along with multiple other foods simply reduce or regulate inflammation which is profoundly beneficial as we have learned that inflammation almost always goes overboard and can easily go haywire. Many inflammatory problems can be reduced or even fully resolved just by modifying your diet and incorporating as many anti-inflammatory foods as you can. As an added benefit, many of these healthy foods can be delicious additions to your diet and most provide more benefits than fighting inflammation.

Other Causes of Inflammation

We know that injury will prompt an immune response and that there are multiple inflammatory diseases, but there are many other triggers for inflammation. Some can cause acute inflammation repeatedly, which can cause repetitive damage and healing leading to scarring, while others can cause constant chronic inflammation that can weaken tissues and even cause wounds inside the body.

Poor gut health is closely related to diet, but worth mentioning as the effect on inflammation in the body is so profound. Your gut is your barrier to the outside world. When the lining of the **gut becomes compromised and intestinal permeability becomes an issue, the body's immune and inflammatory responses are fired up** to deal with digested food cells and foreign bodies that find their way into the bloodstream.

A **lack of sleep** leads to an elevation in inflammatory markers[3].

Chronic stress can be associated with inflammation through the imbalance it can cause in the endocrine system, particularly its effect on adrenaline and cortisol. The fight or flight is another process that is designed to help us in short bursts, but when stress becomes constant or prolonged, the body's endocrine can be thrown out of balance. One effect is inflammation.

Something that people may not associate directly with inflammation is an allergy. **Allergies are an immune response** to something usually harmless that the body views as a dangerous invader. A runny nose is brought on by the excess fluid build-up that enters the nostrils in an attempt to corral the invading pathogens and the redness and itching are caused by the rapid release of histamine. Allergies cause an acute reaction, but some people with multiple allergies or seasonal allergies are often subjected to several acute reactions throughout the day. Allergies are often treated with anti-histamines, but sometimes steroids are used, which work by suppressing the whole immune system.

Being overweight or obese is linked with countless, life threatening diseases from diabetes to heart disease, now we can add chronic inflammation to the list of problems associated with obesity. Recent research has shown that fat, particularly internal abdominal fat, is more than just stored energy. It is in fact, more like a hormone secreting organ than anything else. A little fat is necessary and provides needed hormones and padding for organs, but too much fat produces chemicals that cause inflammation. As individual fat cells swell to great size, the body can begin to target them as threats because large amounts of fat are constantly being attacked by the body's inflammatory response. So, being obese means that your fat is sending out inflammation to other parts of your body while also being attacked. Inflammation can also lead to insulin resistance, which will contribute to more weight gain. Inflammation is one of the reasons why stopping and reversing obesity can be so difficult.

While we often don't think we have it, persistent infections and parasites can stay with you for months or years and cause continued inflammation. These pathogens or parasites are the right things for your inflammatory response to target, but for some reason or another they just can't get rid of them. Parasites often move, making it difficult for the body to section off the parasite and because infections sometimes don't cause high fevers which allows them to move around the body and cause systemic inflammation. The rate of people infected by parasites can be surprising, even in more developed countries. Symptoms of chronic infections or parasites can vary wildly from heart attack to blindness or can have no symptoms at all, but inflammation is still working and slowly degrading parts of your body.

How you live your life can have far more of an impact on chronic inflammation than you may think. Many studies have shown that an inactive lifestyle allows low-level inflammation to affect the entire body causing a double whammy effect of stimulating weight gain just through the inflammatory processes that causes a build-up of inflammatory fat. Even a light exercise schedule can go a long way to reducing this chronic inflammation, but many people still don't find the time to become healthy and the chronic inflammation slowly begins to damage multiple body tissues.

So, if you exercise, you can reverse all of the inflammatory action of a sedentary lifestyle and prevent inflammatory fat from building up, but, if you are addicted to exercise you need to be careful that you do not over train. Even basic exercise causes some inflammation, but this is moderate and acute. Over working your body can cause it to have a difficult time healing from the low level inflammation and continued **overtraining can compound the inflammation** and lead to a runaway cycle of chronic inflammation resulting in diminishing strength and endurance.

Stress is accepted as part of life in the modern world and some people think that the more successful you want to be, the more stress you will have to endure. Stress causes multiple problems, but one of the more recently studied **effects of stress is its role in inflammation**. While normal inflammatory response involves immune cells being transported outside of the blood vessel before doing their inflammatory work, stress will pre-activate these cells to do their inflammatory work without being transported to a trigger spot requiring inflammation. This causes systemic inflammation that can vary based on stress levels, but also alters your body chemistry as your body attempts to regulate inflammation that has no specific target.

Signs You Might be Inflamed

Chronic inflammation can be hard to pin down to specific systems since it can be temporary and low level, making it a fairly nebulous state. Whilst some people could certainly be chronically inflamed without ever noticing the symptoms, you could also present some of these symptoms *without* suffering from chronic inflammation, making it difficult to be certain on.

Having said that, some of things you might look out for

are nasal congestion, water retention, acne flare ups or excessively oily skin, lethargy, excessive stress or tiredness and flare ups in any symptoms related to the inflammatory conditions mentioned previously, like joint paint or red and inflamed skin.

Speak to your doctor if you are worried about chronic inflammation. A test that picks up markers of inflammation in the body like the C-reactive protein can confirm whether or not chronic inflammation is an issue for you, and you can discuss the best course of treatment with your doctor.

THE ANTI-INFLAMMATORY DIET

So, now you know more about inflammation than 99% of the population, including why it's important, but often prolonged and dangerous in the modern environment.

The next question then is – what can I do the fight chronic inflammation, keep myself free from the myriad of related conditions and maximize my health?

The overarching principle is pretty simple: *Exclude factors from your life that promote inflammation, Include factors into your lifestyle that fight inflammation.*

The anti-inflammatory diet is one of the most effective tools for fighting inflammation:

Remove Foods That Promote Inflammation

Include Anti-Inflammatory Foods

Sounds simple right, but what are these factors? We'll dig in below

What to Remove

- **Gluten products** – including wheat and other foods that contain gluten like spelt, barley and rye. This includes foods like bread, pasta, beer, flour, and breaded foods (even whole grain versions)
- **Trans fats** – Partially hydrogenated vegetable oils are being phased out but can still be found in processed foods like frozen pizzas, fried foods, cakes, cookies, margarine & spreads, pie, ready-to-use frosting and coffee creamers. Avoid these.
- **Omega-6 rich Vegetable/Seed Oils** – Sunflower, Corn, Flaxseed, Safflower, Cottonseed, Grapeseed, Flax, walnut and peanut oils are all high in inflammatory omega-6 fatty acids and should be avoided.
- **Sugary foods** – Sweets, treats, cereals and refined sugars should be reduced to keep blood sugar spikes to a minimum.
- **Refined carbohydrates** – Also cause blood sugar spikes and so should be avoided. You will mostly have this covered by removing wheat and gluten products like

bread, pasta and cereal, but beware white rice and noodles can have a similar effect.

What to Include

● **A variety of vegetables** - Vegetables contain anti-oxidants and other natural compounds that will help reduce inflammation. Leafy green vegetables, dark-colored vegetables like red cabbage & beets and cruciferous vegetables are all great at fighting inflammation.

● **Fruit** – Certain fruit are great at modulating inflammation and are low in sugar, like most types of berries, cherries, figs, grapefruit, apples & pears, and apricots & peaches. High-sugar fruit like melon, pineapple, mango and papayas can be enjoyed in moderation.

● **Oily fish** – is a fantastic source of the potent anti-inflammatory omega-3 fatty acid. Mackerel, tuna are all oily fish. You could even consider supplementing with cod liver oil to boost your omega-3 intake.

● **Meat and eggs** – A variety of beef, lamb, pork, poultry and eggs are some of the least inflammatory foods you can go for. However, factory farmed animals raised in stressful conditions and/or with poor diets make unhealthier food – so free-range, grass fed, pasture raised animals will produce the healthiest and most anti-inflammatory foods and are the best choice.

● **Nuts and seeds** – contain a diverse amount of nutrients and other chemical constituents and can reduce markers of inflammation[4].

Personal Choice

- **Milk** – This one's a bit more personal. Many find they are ok drinking cow's milk, whereas some find they do better avoiding milk altogether due to some level of lactose intolerance. The best way to gauge your tolerance is to cut cow's milk out of your diet for 2-4 weeks and the reintroduce it to see if there are any noticeable side effects. If you're not sure, goats milk or low-lactose are good alternatives.

- **Other Dairy (Cheese, Yoghurt etc.)** – Proper cheese and yoghurt are both fermented which reduces the level of lactose, meaning most people better tolerate them. Natural yoghurt also contains beneficial bacteria, which are good anti-inflammatories.

Quick Tip – The Nightshades
Although a variety of richly colored fruit and vegetables should be dietary stalwarts in your new anti-inflammatory lifestyle, be aware of the nightshade family – <u>tomatoes, potatoes and eggplant</u>. These contain the compound solanine, which for some people can evoke pain and the related inflammatory response.

Other Lifestyle Factors to Consider

Gut health – The wholesome approach to nutrition outlined above will remove problematic inflammatory foods from the diet but if have some degree of intestinal permeability then further nutritional support will be needed and your best option is to get a gut permeability test* or consult your local naturopath or dietician for further advice.

Sleep – Aim for 6-8 hours of sleep per night. Reducing your amount of late night screen time or downloading the flux app can help with resetting your body clock. If you find getting to sleep particularly difficult you could also consider getting a blue therapy light for use in the morning to reset your body clock or experiment with mindfulness based approach to insomnia**.

Stress - Steps should be taken minimize prolonged and chronic stress. Don't underestimate the importance of downtime for your health - relaxation time away from screens and work is important to give the body and mind recovery periods. Many find light exercise outdoors useful for relaxing like going for walks, cycling, or playing Frisbee or catch. Many also report relaxation exercises and mindfulness exercises like mindfulness based cognitive therapy (MBCT) or mindfulness based stress reduction (MBCR) as useful tools in changing their reaction to stressful events in their life. There are also a couple of dietary supplements worth noting when it comes to beating stress – both L-Theanine and Phosphatidyl Serine have anti-stress properties.

Exercise – Whilst frequent exercise generally leads to a decrease in inflammation, it's important to have recovery periods between training sessions. The body's reaction to most forms of exercise an acute inflammatory response – as anyone who's completed a particularly intense sprint session or Olympic lifting session will know the next day from the ache in their muscles.

The body needs periods of recovery, particularly after intense workouts, to avoid a state of constant exercise induced inflammation. Remember to schedule rest days between your workouts (this is particularly true for sports where a high volume of training is required e.g. long distance endurance training and marathons.)

* Like the mannitol/sorbitol test or the PEG test
** For example, see *The Sleep Book* by Guy Meadows

Top 5 Anti-Inflammatory Foods

The guidelines above provide a great approach to treating inflammation through diet and lifestyle changes, but here are a few foods that can bolster your anti-inflammatory efforts

1. Turmeric

Turmeric is famed for its therapeutic effect, part of which is due to curcumin, one of the anti-inflammatories it contains. For extra brownie points try consuming it with some black pepper or try a fermented version – both methods increase the bioavailability or curcumin.

2. Oily Fish

Fish like mackerel, salmon and sardines are naturally oily so they're a great choice for boosting your omega-3 fatty acid intake. Supplemental cod liver oil is also available in capsule form if you don't think you're getting enough omega-3.

3. Cruciferous Vegetables

This family of vegetables includes cabbage, broccoli, cauliflower and brussel sprouts, which are rich in helpful compounds like Sulforaphane.

4. Berries

You probably don't need much encouragement from me to eat more berries – they're delicious and they already have a great reputation as being a 'superfood' group. They're relatively low in sugar and contain a good array of micronutrients and phytochemicals. The only problem is that their high surface area means they're easily contaminated by pesticides, so be sure to wash them thoroughly or buy organic.

6. Fermented Foods

Foods that have been fermented – i.e. broken down by the naturally occurring bacteria they contain, like sauerkraut, kefir and kombucha – are a source of benficial bacteria. Considering there are 10 bacteria cells for every 1 human cell in your body, it's important to include fermented foods in your diet to ensure a healthy micro biome. Supplements are also available containing freeze-dried bacterial cultures.

Heath Easton

Part 2: Recipes

BREAKFAST

Morning Breakfast Green Smoothie

Prep time: 5 minutes
Servings: 1

Ingredients

2 cups of fresh spinach leaves
½ cup of almond milk
2 scoops of vanilla protein powder or fresh egg (optional)
1 Tbsp of almond butter or peanut butter
a handful of ice
1 tsp of dark cocoa powder, unsweetened
½ avocado
1 ripe banana

Instructions

- Place all the ingredients in a blender and process until smooth.

Spiced Kale Scramble

Prep time: 5 minutes
Cooking time: 7 minutes
Servings: 1

Ingredients
2 eggs
1 cup of fresh kale, chopped
1½ tsp of turmeric
1 tsp of garlic powder
1 Tbsp of butter
Salt and pepper to taste

Instructions
- Whisk eggs in a small bowl, set aside.
- Heat butter in a large skillet over medium-high heat, then add the chopped kale and cook until kale wilts. Add the eggs.
- Stir in turmeric powder and season with garlic powder, salt and pepper and continue cooking until eggs are set.
- Serve warm.

Natural Goat Yoghurt with Berries

Prep time: 2 minutes
Servings: 1

Ingredients
1 pot natural goat yoghurt
A couple of handfuls of fresh berries or sliced fruit
1 tsp natural honey
Optional: Crushed or flaked nuts

Instructions
- Pour your chosen selection of fruit, berries and nuts into the yoghurt. Drizzle with honey, and serve.

Eggs Benedict On Grain-Free Waffles

Prep time: 15 minutes
Cooking time: 15 minutes
Servings: 4

Ingredients

Waffles
3 eggs
¾ cup raw cashew butter
3 Tbsp of almond milk
2 tsp of bacon fat or ghee, melted
¼ tsp of garlic, minced
¼ tsp of salt
¾ tsp of baking soda
3 Tbsp of coconut flour
1 piece bacon, roughly chopped
2 chives, chopped

Hollandaise Sauce
2 egg yolks
¼ cup of unsalted butter or ghee, melted
2 tsp of lemon juice
¼ tsp of salt
1/8 tsp Paprika or Cayenne (optional)

To Serve

4 savory waffles

4 slices of ham, cooked

4 eggs, poached

¼ cup of Hollandaise sauce

Chives for garnish

Instructions

Process Waffles and Benedict

- Preheat your waffle maker.

- Whisk the eggs together with cashew butter, almond milk, bacon fat and garlic, using a stand mixer or handheld mixer.

- In a small bowl, combine salt, baking soda and coconut flour.

- Add in the flour mixture to the egg mixture and beat for 30 seconds or until the batter is well combined, scraping the bottom of bowl to get all the sticky cashew butter.

- Use your hands to combine the chopped bacon and chives into the batter.

- Cook the waffles in your waffle maker, according to manufacturer's instructions.

- Set aside the cooked waffles, but keep it warm until the Benedict is ready for assembling.

Process Hollandaise Sauce

- Pour very hot water into the blender to clean it, then discard the water and dry the blender thoroughly.

- Combine egg yolks, lemon juice and paprika in the clean blender.

- Turn on the blender on the lowest setting, and slowly pour in the hot melted butter and blend for about 30 seconds or until sauce thickens and well combined.

- Remember that the sauce will continue to thicken as it cools; if it gets too thick, warm it over low heat (1 minutes) or microwave (about 10 seconds) until it becomes runny again.

- Too much heat will make your egg like scrambled eggs and your butter will curdle, so be careful.

- To serve, layer the waffles, ham slices, poached egg and drizzle with hollandaise sauce and garnish with a few chives.

Chorizo Tomato Frittata

Prep time: 10 minutes
Cooking time: 10 minutes
Servings: 3

Ingredients
6 eggs
½ cup of goat's cream
1 chorizo sausage, peeled
1 yellow onion, chopped
½ large zucchini, diced
1 Roma tomato, thinly sliced
1 garlic clove, peeled and finely diced
½ tsp of sweet paprika
1 tsp ghee or 2 Tbsp olive oil
Fresh basil
Salt and pepper

Instructions
- Halved the chorizo sausage. Slice one half into small disks and diced the other half.
- Heat a little ghee or 1 Tbsp of olive oil in a large skillet over medium heat.
- Fry the chorizo disks on both sides then transfer to a plate lined with paper towels.
- Add a little more ghee or olive oil to the same skillet, then sauté the onions, garlic and zucchini.

- Add the diced chorizo sausage. Continue cooking over medium heat until sausage softened.
- Stir in paprika.
- Meanwhile, in a bowl, whisk 5 eggs, cream and ½ tsp of salt together. Mix well.
- Spread the onion/chorizo mixture evenly in the skillet, then pour the egg mixture over the surface.
- Arrange tomato slices and fried chorizo slices on top.
- Make a well in the center of the egg mixture and crack the last egg to the center, gently, making sure to keep the yolk intact.
- Cover the skillet and cook till set, then uncover and cook for 1 more minute.
- Transfer cooked omelette on a serving platter and sprinkle on top with ground black pepper and fresh basil leaves just before serving.

Make-Ahead Creole Casserole

Prep time: 15 minutes
Cooking time: 30 minutes
Servings: 5

Ingredients
4-5 Andouille sausages (about 12oz)
½ large bell pepper
½ jalapeno, chopped
½ yellow onion, chopped
8 eggs
2 Tbsp of hot sauce
2 Tbsp of Worcestershire sauce

Instructions
- Preheat oven to 350°F/180°C. Prepare an 8x8-inch baking pan.
- Heat a non-stick pan and cook the sausage until brown, then add peppers, onions, and sauté until onions are soft. Turn off the heat and set aside the sautéed mixture to cool.
- Whisk the eggs directly on a baking pan, together with hot sauce and Worcestershire sauce.
- Add the sautéed sausage mixture into the beaten egg mixture and whisk again to combine.
- Bake in preheated oven for about 30 minutes or until eggs set.
- Cut it into squares and arrange neatly in a container.

- Refrigerate, uncovered until it cools, then cover the container.

LUNCH

Nicoise Salad

Prep time: 10 minutes
Cooking time: 20 minutes
Servings: 4

Ingredients

12-15 baby potatoes, unpeeled and thickly sliced
2 Tbsp of olive oil
2 tsp of olive oil
4 eggs
2 Tbsp of capers, rinsed
1.8oz Sun Blush or sun dried tomatoes in oil, finely chopped
½ red onion, thinly sliced
3.5oz baby spinach
2 x cans (~15oz each) yellow fin tuna steak in spring water, drained

Instructions

- Preheat oven to 200°C/fan 180°C/gas 6.
- Season the potatoes with 2 tsp oil and salt+pepper.
- Arrange potatoes on a large baking pan and roast, stirring halfway until crisp and golden brown, about 20 minutes.
- Meanwhile, boil the eggs depending on how you liked them cooked.
- Submerge eggs into a bowl of cold water, then peel away the shells and cut each egg in half.
- Whisk the remaining oil in a salad bowl, together with red wine vinegar, capers and chopped tomatoes.

- Stir in the onions, spinach, tuna and potatoes. Toss everything together.
- Garnish salad with boiled eggs and serve immediately.

Greek Salad

Prep time: 10 minutes
Cooking time: 10 minutes
Servings: 8

Ingredients

3 cucumbers, seeded and sliced
1 ½ cups of Feta cheese, crumbled (made from goat's milk)
1 cup of black olives, pitted and sliced
3 cups of Roma tomatoes, diced
1/3 cup of diced, oil packed sun-dried tomatoes (drained, oil reserved)
½ red onion, sliced

Instructions

- In a large salad bowl, combine cucumbers, feta cheese, olives, Roma tomatoes, sun-dried tomatoes, 2 tablespoons reserved sun-dried tomato oil, and red onion. Toss together gently till combined.
- Chill just before serving.

Cinnamon Mackerel Curry

Prep time: 10 minutes
Cooking time: 25 minutes
Servings: 2

Ingredients
1 can mackerel (15oz)
1 tomato, chopped
1 Tbsp of curry powder
2 Tbsp of black pepper powder
¼ tsp of turmeric powder
1 cinnamon stick
1 onion, thinly sliced
1 Tbsp of garlic, crushed
2 cups of water
Salt to taste
2 Tbsp of olive oil
3oz coconut milk
1 Tbsp of fenugreek seeds
1 tsp of black mustard seeds
10 curry leaves, finely chopped
1 green chili or capsicum, sliced lengthwise
½ tsp red chili powder

Instructions
- Heat the oil in a pan and add the black mustard seeds, sautéing until they start to pop (about 5 minutes)

- Stir in the onion, curry powder, garlic, pepper, turmeric, curry leaves, chili, fenugreek seeds and red chili powder. Sauté over a medium-high heat whilst stirring continuously for 5 minutes.
- Add in chopped tomato and cinnamon stick and sauté for 2 more minutes.
- Drain the can of mackerel (reserving the liquid) and add the fish into the mixture, stirring frequently.
- Slightly break fish into but size pieces.
- Fish breaks easily so you need to cut into bite sized chunks. Too small chunks will make it mushy.
- Add in the saved fish liquid and 2 cup of water.
- Mix in the coconut milk and adjust the seasonings, adding salt and pepper if necessary.
- Lower the heat and simmer for 10 minutes.
- Serve hot over rice with a side dish of sautéed vegetables.

Chipotle-Lime Prawn Salsa with Avocado Mash

Prep time: 10 minutes
Cooking time: 10 minutes
Servings: 4

Ingredients
1 medium ripe avocado
Juice from ¼ lemon
12-15 large prawns, cooked and peeled
1 tomato, diced
2 sprigs coriander or parsley, finely chopped
Juice from 1 lime
1 Tbsp red onion, finely chopped
2 Tbsp chipotle chili sauce

Instructions
- Peel the avocado and discard the skin. Slice into cubes and mash together with lemon juice.
- Spread mashed avocado evenly on a serving platter.
- Cut each prawns into three chunks and combine with tomato, chopped coriander or parsley, lime juice, chopped onion and chili sauce. Toss to combine. Refrigerate until ready to serve.
- When ready to serve, topped avocado mashed with prawn salsa with a drizzle of extra chili sauce if you like it hot.
- Serve with lettuce wraps.

Sirloin Salad with Balsamic Vinaigrette

Prep time: 15 minutes
Cooking time: 5 minutes
Servings: 2-4

Ingredients

Salad
6 cups of spinach
½ cup of bacon, cooked and crumbled
½ cup of goat's cheese, crumbled
½ cup of flaked almonds
½ cup of dried cranberries
½ cup of cherry tomatoes, diced
½ cup red onion, thinly sliced
½ lb grass-fed sirloin, cooked to your liking and sliced

Dressing
¼ cup of balsamic vinegar
2 garlic cloves, peeled
Salt and pepper to taste
¾ cup extra virgin olive oil

Instructions
- Place the spinach on the bottom of a large salad bowl.
- Place a portion of bacon on one side of the bowl, a portion of goat cheese, a portion of almonds, a portion of

cranberries, a portion of tomatoes and a portion of red onions. Arrange them side by side around the salad bowl, leaving a space in the middle.

- Put the sliced beef in the middle portion of a salad bowl.

- For the dressing, in a bowl of your food processor, combine the balsamic vinegar, garlic, salt and pepper and process until the mixture is smooth and well combined.

- Add the olive oil slowly while and continue to process while your dressing emulsifies.

- Serve the dressing with your salad, either on side or to drizzle on top.

Chicken Liver Pâté

Prep time: 10 minutes
Cooking time: 20 minutes
Makes 3-4 ramekins

Ingredients
1 lb Chicken liver
1 small onion (or 1/2 of a large onion)
0.5 c red wine
3 cloves garlic, crushed
1 tsp Dijon mustard
1 sprig Fresh rosemary
2 sprigs Fresh thyme
1 Tbsp Fresh lemon juice
0.5 c + 4 Tbsp Butter or clarified butter
Sea salt and cracked black pepper

Instructions
- Finely chop the onion. Remove the white connective parts of the liver with a knife, then coarsely chop. Sauté both in a pan along with a couple of Tbsp of butter over a medium heat, until the livers are browned and the onions tender.
- Add wine, garlic, mustard, herbs and lemon juice and cook uncovered until most of the liquid has gone.
- Blend the mixture in a food pressure for 2-3 minutes until you've reached a smooth consistency. Melt half a cup

of butter in the microwave and slowly add it to the mixture whilst blending until all the butter is added and you've reached the consistency of a smooth pate.

- Season well with salt and pepper, then transfer to ramekins or a shallow dish.

- Finally, pour a small amount of butter over the top of the pate to form a seal, and allow to cool and set in the refrigerator.

- Serve with sticks of carrot, cucumber of bell pepper.

Sticky Portuguese Churrasqueira Chicken Wings

Prep time: 10 minutes
Cooking time: 12 minutes
Servings: 12 to 14 wings

Ingredients
12-14 chicken wings
Coconut oil or ghee for cooking

Marinade:
2 large garlic cloves, grated
Zest of 1 lemon
Juice of ½ lemon
2 tsp of tomato paste
2/3 tsp of ground coriander seeds
2/3 tsp of onion powder
1 ½ Tbsp Tamari (wheat free) soy sauce
2 tsp of coconut oil (melted)
2/3 tsp of sea salt

Instructions
- Wash and rinse the chicken wings, then pat dry with paper towels.
- In a large mixing bow, combine grated garlic, lemon zest, lemon juice, tomato paste, coriander seeds, onion powder, tamari soy sauce, coconut oil and salt. Mix well to combine.

- Coat chicken wings with marinade mixture, tossing evenly to coat each wings thoroughly with the marinade.

- Marinate wings ideally for 1 hour, but you can proceed to cooking process if pressed for time.

- Heat a large skillet with 1 Tbsp of coconut oil or ghee over medium-high heat.

- Place chicken wings on hot oil, skin side up. Fry wings in batches as we do not want to overcrowd the skillet.

- Fry wings over medium-high heat for about 6 minutes; cover the skillet during the last 2 minutes of cooking time.

- Covering the pan helps to keep the wings nice and soft.

- Alternatively, you can bake this in the preheated oven, 395°F/200°C for 40 minutes.

- Serve with some steamed green vegetables or salad and a sliced lemon on the side.

DINNER

Curry Meatballs with Liver

Prep time: 10 minutes
Cooking time: 30 minutes
Makes 20 meatballs

For the Meatballs
0.5 lb Liver (or heart, tongue, kidney etc.)
1.5 lb Ground meat (pork, beef, or a combination)
1 Egg
3 Garlic cloves
1 Tbsp curry powder
Salt and Pepper
Large handful fresh parsley
Small handful fresh mint leaves

For the Sauce
3 Tbsp butter
1 Onion
4 Garlic cloves
Large knob of root ginger
2 t Ground coriander
2 t Ground cumin
1 t Curry powder
1 can Chopped tomatoes
1 can Coconut milk
3 Carrots
Salt and Pepper

Instructions

- Peel and finely chop the garlic, ginger and onion and sauté in in a little coconut oil in a pot over a medium heat. When the onion is beginning to soften, add the spices.

- Allow the spices to become fragrant for a minute or two then add the canned tomatoes and cook for 5 minutes.

- Meanwhile, peel and chop the carrot into 0.5 inch rounds and add to the pan along with the coconut milk. Allow to simmer on a low heat whilst you make the meatballs.

- Add the meatball ingredients to a food processor and process until well blended. Use your hands to form 20 meatballs.

- Heat some coconut oil in a pan and brown the meatballs for 3-4 minutes on each side.

- Pour the coconut sauce over the meatballs and continue to simmer for 10-15 minutes more, or until the sauce has thickened and the meatballs are cooked through.

Turmeric and Lime Salmon

Prep time: 10 minutes + 20 minutes marinating
Cooking time: 10 minutes
Servings: 2-3

Ingredients
2-3 salmon fillets (6oz each)
½ tsp of white pepper, coarsely ground
2 Tbsp of fresh lime juice (½ large lime)
1 red chili, deseeded and finely chopped
1 Tbsp of fish sauce
1 Tbsp of tamari (wheat free) soy sauce
½ small onion, finely chopped
1 Tbsp lime leaf, chopped (or lime zest)
Olive oil (to brush on griddle)
6 stalks spring onions, trimmed and sliced in half lengthwise

For the rice
150g brown rice
1 tsp olive oil
300ml hot vegetable stock (not too salty or strongly made up)
½ tsp chopped lime leaf OR lime zest

Instructions
- Prepare a dish that is large enough to fit the fish snugly.

- Combine ground white pepper, lime juice, red chili, fish sauce, tamari soy sauce, chopped onion and lime leaf in a prepared dish. Mix well to combine.

- Place the fish in the marinating mixture, turning a few time to coat the fish with marinade, then cover with plastic wrap and marinate for about 20 minutes to let the flavors develop.

- When ready, remove the fish from the marinade (reserving it for later), brush the fish with a little oil and place on a griddle pan or the oiled surface of your hob-top griddle pan along with the spring onions.

- Cooking time varies, depending on the thickness of the fish – usually 4-5 minutes each side. The fish is cooked when it flakes easily when prick with a fork. It can be a little tricky, so test using your own method.

- Transfer fish and spring onion to a serving platter and serve with rice or steamed green vegetables.

Lemon, Garlic and Paprika Grilled Sardines

Prep time: 10 minutes + 10 minutes marinating
Cooking time: 10 minutes
Servings: 2-4

Ingredients

3 medium garlic cloves (1 Tbsp), finely minced
¼ cup of extra virgin olive oil
¼ cup of fresh lemon juice
1 tsp of smoked Spanish paprika
½ tsp of freshly ground black pepper
1 lb fresh sardines, cleaned, scaled and gutted
Fine sea salt or kosher salt
2 Tbsp of fresh parsley, chopped
Lemon wedges (for garnish)

Instructions

- In a small bowl, whisk together garlic, olive oil, lemon juice, paprika and black pepper.
- Prepare a shallow baking dish that will fit the fish snugly in single layer.
- Arrange the fish in a baking dish and pour sauce mixture over the fish, turning the fish several times to ensure they are coated evenly with the marinade. Pour the marinade inside fish cavity.
- Marinate fish for 30 minutes.
- Meanwhile, prepare and preheat your gas or charcoal

grill.

- If using the oven, set the gas grill to the highest setting and preheat for 10 minutes.

- Wash and clean the grilling grates and brush with oil.

- Discard the marinade.

- Grill the sardines over the hot coals until well-charred, about 3 minutes. Flip the sardines and grill the other side until charred and cooked through, about 3 minutes longer.

-Place the sardines on a plate and sprinkle with salt.

- Garnish with chopped fresh parsley and lemon wedges.

Soulful Chicken Soup

Prep time: 15 minutes
Cooking time: 15 minutes
Servings: 2

Ingredients

¼ whole cooked chicken on the bone
1 tsp of olive oil
2 tsp of lemongrass, minced
2 tsp of ginger, grated
3 sprigs of spring onions, sliced
4 cups chicken broth
2 cups Chinese broccoli, trimmed and sliced into 1-inch length
½ head broccoli, trimmed into florets
1 bag (40z) baby spinach leaves
Sea salt and pepper to taste

To serve
Extra spring onions (green part only)
Chicken meat (from step 1)
Chili powder, if using

Instructions

- Remove the chicken skin and set aside. Separate meat from the bones. Set aside the bones.
- Heat oil over medium-heat using a large heavy pan, and

sauté the lemongrass, ginger, garlic and spring onions, until fragrant, about 1 minute.

- Add the broth and the bones and skins of chicken. Bring to a boil.

- Lower the heat and cook to a gentle simmer for about 5 minutes.

- Discard the bones and skins from the stock.

- To the stock, add in the Chinese broccoli and broccoli florets and cook for further 2 minutes.

- Add the baby spinach and add salt and pepper to taste, adding seasonings as necessary.

- Serve the soup hot topped with shredded chicken meat, dust with chili powder (if using) and extra spring onions.

Beef, Bacon and Butternut Squash Chili

Prep time: 10 minutes
Cooking time: 45 minutes
Servings: 4

Ingredients
1 ½ lbs butternut squash, peeled, seeded and cubed
6 slices of bacon
1 lb ground beef
1 red onion, diced
3 jalapenos, diced
2 cloves garlic, finely chopped
5 roma tomatoes, diced
¼ cup of cider vinegar
1 tsp of sea salt
1 tsp of oregano
½ tsp of cumin
½ tsp of cayenne
2 Tbsp of coconut oil, melted

Instructions
- Preheat oven to 400°F/205°C.
- Combine the cubed butternut squash and coconut oil in a roasting pan and roast in a preheated oven for about 30 minutes or until squash are tender.
- Meanwhile, heat a large heavy skillet over medium-high heat and cook the bacon until crisp. Transfer the bacon

into a plate and set aside to cool, leaving the bacon grease in a skillet.

- Add the bison or beef to the bacon grease in the skillet and cook until it changes in color and is no longer pink.

- Add in the diced onion, garlic and diced jalapenos and cook until the onions are soft.

- Season with salt, oregano, cumin and cayenne and continue cooking, stirring frequently for 1 minute.

- Crumble or slice the bacon and add to the skillet.

- Stir in the tomatoes with their juice and the apple cider vinegar.

- Lower the heat and simmer until sauce thickens, about 30 minutes.

- To serve, place the chili in a bowl, topped with cooked butternut squash.

- Dust with cocoa or cinnamon powder (optional). Serve with cauliflower rice or steamed veggies.

Thai Shellfish Soup

Prep time: 2 minutes
Cooking time: 15 minutes
Servings: 4

Ingredients
3 cups bone broth or water
Small piece of root ginger
8 oz. white mushrooms, sliced
1 bag (~10oz) Frozen fruits de mer (mix of mussels, prawns, scallops, squid rings)
2 cans (13oz each) Coconut milk
3 T Red or green Thai curry paste
2 Limes
2 Scallions
Optional: 2 T Dried wakame or kombu seaweed

Instructions
- Peel and finely slice the ginger and sauté over a medium head in a pot with a little coconut oil or butter for 3 minutes.
- Add the curry paste and stir for a couple of minutes until it becomes fragrant.
- Roughly chop the mushrooms and add to the pot along with the coconut milk, broth, seaweed and shellfish.
- Bring to the boil and simmer for 10 minutes. Meanwhile, finely chop the scallions and juice the limes.

- Add the lime juice to the soup then pour into bowls. Garnish with the chopped scallion and serve.

Baked Pork & Apple Meatballs

Prep time: 15 minutes
Cooking time: 30 minutes
Servings: 8

Ingredients

2 ½ lbs ground pork
2 apples, peeled and finely diced
2 garlic cloves, finely minced
2 Tbsp of onion powder
2 Tbsp of ground sage
1 tsp of white pepper
1 tsp of cinnamon
1 ½ tsp of sea salt

Instructions

- Preheat oven to 425°F/215°C.
- Line the bottom of 1 or 2 rimmed baking sheets with parchment paper.
- In a large bowl, combine minced garlic (or use 1 Tbsp of garlic powder), onion powder, white pepper, ground sage and cinnamon. Mix well
- Combine the spices mixture with the ground pork. Use your hands to mix the spices into the pork, then add the diced apples and some salt and mix it all together.
- Form 30-40 meatballs (about 1oz each) and arrange them evenly on the prepared baking sheet.
- Bake in the preheated oven for about 30 minutes or until

meatballs turns golden brown.

- Serve meatballs with mashed cauliflower or your favorite side dish.

SIDE DISHES + SNACKS

Best-Ever Braised Cabbage

Prep time: 10 minutes
Cooking time: 1 hour
Servings: 4-6

Ingredients

2 Tbsp of lard, ghee or bacon grease, melted
1 medium head (2 lbs) green (savoy) cabbage
1 large red or yellow onion, peeled and thickly sliced
2 carrots, peeled and cut into ¼ inch rounds
¼ cup meat stock or water
¼ cup lard, ghee or bacon grease
Coarse sea salt and fresh ground pepper
Aged balsamic vinegar

Instructions

- Preheat oven to 325°F/165°C. Place the rack in the middle of the oven.
- Grease a 13x9-inch baking pan with melted fat (lard, ghee or bacon grease).
- Cut cabbage into 6-8 wedges, keeping the core attached for the cabbage to stay intact during cooking time.
- Arrange cabbage wedges in a single layer on a greased baking pan. Distribute the onions and carrots evenly and drizzle the stock or water and the melted fat.
- Add salt and pepper to taste.
- Cover the baking pan with foil and put inside the oven to

bake for 1 hour, undisturbed.

- After one hour, slightly open the foil cover and flip the wedges gently. Cover again with foil and bake for another 1 hour or until cabbage is fork tender.

- Transfer the cabbage to a clean container to cool.

- Refrigerate until you want to eat. It can be refrigerated for up to 4 days.

- When ready to eat or serve, preheat oven to 425°F/215°C and bake the cabbage until browned, about 15 minutes.

- Serve immediately with a generous drizzle of balsamic vinegar.

Quick and Easy Green Salad

Prep time: 5-10 minutes
Servings: 3-4

Ingredients
1 large bag of pre-cut kale
Extra virgin olive oil
Juice of 1 lemon
1 cup of Parmesan cheese or feta cheese, pre-grated
1 tsp of red pepper flakes
Salt to taste

Instructions
- Wash kale, then pick the leaves and tear large leaves into manageable pieces. Discard the stems.
- Place the leaves into a large bowl and drizzle with a bit of olive oil, just enough to coat all the leaves.
- Massage the oiled leaves, using your hands, until you feel that the volume of the leaves reduce by 1/3, that is the time to add the lemon juice, salt, red pepper flakes and Parmesan or feta cheese. Toss to combine.
- Taste and adjust the seasonings, according to your preference.
- Refrigerate until ready to serve.

Halloumi, Pomegranate Seeds and Cherries

Prep time: 10 minutes
Cooking time: 5 minutes
Servings: 2-4

Ingredients

One (225g/ 8oz) packet Halloumi cheese
1 Tbsp of olive oil
1 cup of hummus
1 tsp of coriander, finely chopped
Pinch of chili powder
Seeds of ½ pomegranate
10 fresh cherries, halved and pitted
¼ cup of flat leaf parsley, finely chopped
2 Tbsp of lemon juice

Instructions

- In a small bowl, combine hummus, ground coriander and pinch of chili powder. Mix well.
- Cut halloumi cheese into thin slices.
- Heat oil in a medium skillet, over medium-high heat and fry halloumi cheese on both sides until golden brown. Remove from pan and set aside.
- Spread hummus evenly on a serving platter, topped with slices of fried halloumi cheese.
- Arrange pomegranate seeds and cherries on top and sprinkle with chopped fresh parsley.

- Serve the salad warm with a drizzle of lemon juice.

Prosciutto-Wrapped Asparagus

Prep time: 5 minutes
Cooking time: 10 minutes
Servings: 10

Ingredients
3 bunches of asparagus, stems trimmed 2-inches from the bottom
2 packages (4oz) prosciutto de parma
Sea salt
Freshly ground pepper
2 Tbsp of melted ghee or bacon fat
Aged balsamic vinegar

Instructions
- Prepare the broiler; arrange the rack, 6 inches from the heating element and preheat the broiler over high heat
- Lay the asparagus evenly, in s single layer onto two large baking sheets, then drizzle with melted ghee and add sprinkle with salt and pepper.
- Cut each piece of prosciutto into 3 thin slices lengthwise and wrap each one strip of prosciutto around each asparagus spear.
- Place one tray under a broiler and broil for 5-8 minutes, tossing and turning the spears until prosciutto is crispy and the asparagus tender. Repeat the cooking procedure with the second tray.

- Arrange wrapped asparagus spears on a serving platter with a drizzle of balsamic vinegar.

Turmeric Roasted Cauliflower

Prep time: 10 minutes
Cooking time: 1 hour and 15 minutes
Servings: 2

Ingredients
Half of a large cauliflower, cut into florets
2 tsp of turmeric
2 tsp of salt
2 Tbsp of olive oil

Instructions
- Preheat oven to 350°F/180°C.
- In a bowl, mix together cauliflower florets, turmeric powder, salt and olive oil and toss to combine.
- Spread cauliflower into a baking pan, making sure they are not on top of each other; cover with foil.
- Bake in preheated oven until the cauliflower is tender, about 75 minutes. If you like, remove the after 50-55 minutes to allow the cauliflower to color.

Garlic Roasted Broccoli

Prep time: 10 minutes
Cooking time: 15-20 minutes
Servings: 4

Ingredients

2 heads of broccoli, cut into florets
3 Tbsp of olive oil
5 cloves garlic, minced
1 tsp of salt
½ tsp of ground black pepper
1 tsp of lemon juice
Pinch of red pepper flakes (optional)

Instructions

- Preheat oven to 300°F/150°C.
- In a bowl, combine broccoli florets, olive oil, salt, black pepper and garlic.
- Spread broccoli florets into a baking pan, making sure they are not on top of each other and bake until florets are tender and brown on the edges, about 15 minutes.
- Toss the florets, halfway through baking process and add a dash of red pepper flakes.
- Serve broccoli florets with a squeezed of fresh lemon juice.

DRINKS

Turmeric-Pepper Tea Infusion

Prep time: 10 minutes
Cooking time: 10 minutes
Servings: 4

Ingredients
32oz boiling water
½ Tbsp of turmeric powder
1 Tbsp of fresh ginger, thinly sliced
1 handful cilantro, chopped
1 garlic clove, peeled and crushed
1 Tbsp of olive oil
Juice of 2 lemons
5 whole peppercorns
Juice of 1 orange (or 1 ½ Tbsp honey)

Instructions
- Bring water to a boil.
- Combine turmeric powder, ginger, cilantro, garlic, olive oil, lemon juice, peppercorns and orange juice in a teapot.
- Pour the boiling water on the teapot and let the mixture steep for 5-10 minutes. Strain.
- Serve hot!

Frozen Fruit Smoothie

Prep time: 5 – 10 minutes
Servings: 2

Ingredients

2 cups of frozen watermelon flesh, cut into small chunks
1 cup of frozen pineapple, cut into small chunks
1 orange, peeled, white pith and seeds removed
½ cup of coconut milk
1 ½ cups of coconut water
1 tsp of fresh ginger, grated
½ tsp of turmeric powder
1 tsp of honey (optional)

Instructions

- Place all the ingredients in a blender and blend until smooth and frosty
- Pour the smoothie in a tall glass and serve.

Creamy Coconut Turmeric Tea

Ingredients
1 cup(8oz) Coconut milk
0.5 tsp Turmeric powder
1/2-inch piece Root Ginger, peeled and finely chopped
Dash of cayenne pepper
Dash of black pepper
0.5 tsp Honey or other sweetener
Optional: a small pat of butter, cinnamon, cardamom

Instructions
- Heat the coconut or almond milk in on the stove or microwave.
- Combine the turmeric, ginger, sweetener, cayenne pepper and black pepper in a mug.
- Add a small amount of the coconut milk to the mug and stir the ingredients well to remove any lumps. Add the rest of the warm coconut milk.
- Strain the solids out through a sieve, and enjoy.

DESSERTS

Grain-Free Chocolate Pumpkin Pecan Brownies

Prep time: 15 minutes

Cooking time: 35 minutes

Servings: Makes one 8x8-inch pan of brownies

Ingredients

1 large ripe banana, peeled and cut in half

1 Tbsp of coconut oil, melted

6 Tbsp of pumpkin puree (from a can)

1 cup of fresh kale, chopped

1 can (15oz) of black beans, drained and rinsed

1/3 cup of coconut sugar

1/3 cup of natural honey

6 Tbsp of cocoa powder

a pinch of sea salt

1 tsp cinnamon

1 Tbsp + 1 tsp of pure vanilla extract

¼ cup of oat flour

½ tsp of baking powder

¼ cup pecans, chopped

¼ cup of dark chocolate, cut into chunks

Brownie Topping

3oz dark chocolate bar, melted

Whole Pecans

Instructions

- Preheat oven to 350°F/180°C.
- Prepare an 8x8-inch baking tray, line the bottom with parchment paper and grease with coconut oil.
- Put the banana in a blender or food processor together with melted coconut oil, pumpkin puree, drained beans, coconut sugar and honey. Process until smooth.
- Stir in the cocoa powder, pink salt, cinnamon, vanilla extract, oat flour and baking powder and continue to process until smooth.
- Mix in the chopped pecans and chocolate chunks and fold in gently, then pour the mixture into the prepared tray.
- Spread the brownie mixture evenly in tray and bake for about 35 minutes or until a toothpick inserted in the center comes out clean (Do not over-bake)
- Cut into serving squares and garnish each brownie slice with whole pecan.

Salt Chocolate Pear Wedges

Prep time: 5 minutes
Cooking time: 15 minutes
Servings: 4

Ingredients
½ lemon
4 ripe pears
1 cup of dark chocolate chips
Flaked sea salt

Instructions
- Prepare a baking sheet, line the baking sheet with parchment paper.
- Slice pears into wedges and squeeze the lemon all over the pears Toss to coat the pears with lemon juice. Lemon juice helps to prevent the pears from turning brown.
- Melt the chocolate chips in a double boiler (bain-marie). Whisk chocolate until completely melted; remove from heat.
- Dip pear wedges into the melted chocolate and arrange them in a single layer on the prepared baking sheet. Sprinkle with some flake salt or coarse salt.
- Refrigerate until the chocolate coating hardens, about 15 minutes.
- Serve and enjoy!

Apple Cobbler

Prep time: 10 minutes
Cooking time: 15-20 minutes
Servings: 4

Ingredients
3 Tbsp of butter
1 tsp of lemon juice
2 lbs apples, peeled, cored and chopped
1/3 cup of apple juice concentrates
¼ cup of raisins
½ tsp of vanilla extract
½ tsp of ground cinnamon
¼ tsp of ground ginger
¼ tsp of grated nutmeg

Topping
3 Tbsp of tapioca flour
1 Tbsp of coconut flour
½ stick (2oz) cold butter, cut into small cubes
1 Tbsp of apple juice concentrates

Instructions
- Preheat the broiler and place oven rack in the middle layer of the oven.
- Melt the butter in a medium cast iron skillet over medium-high heat and add in the lemon juice, apples,

apple concentrate, raisins, vanilla, cinnamon, ginger and nutmeg. Stir to combine.

- Continue cooking until the apple juice concentrate has reduced and thickens, about 6 minutes. Turn off heat.

- Meanwhile, prepare the topping by combining tapioca and coconut flour.

- Add the butter into the flour and rub the mixture using your hands to create crumbs. Stir in apple juice slowly.

- Sprinkle this topping mixture on top of cooked apples and broil in the oven until top is golden brown, about 5 to 6 minutes.

The Anti-Inflammatory Diet

Thank You Gift

I want to say Thank You for buying my book so I put together a free gift for you!

This page contains a quick reference guide to gluten, fats and oils is for you to print off and keep handy in the kitchen so visit the link below to get access.

www.BlueBeanPublishing.com/Anti-Inflammatory

Disclaimer/Terms of Use
The Anti-Inflammatory Diet By Heath Easton

Disclaimer and Terms of Use: This document is geared towards providing exact and reliable information in regards to the topic and issue covered. The publication is sold with the idea that the publisher is not required to render accounting, officially permitted, or otherwise, qualified services. If advice is necessary, legal or professional, a practiced individual in the profession should be ordered.

From a Declaration of Principles which was accepted and approved equally by a Committee of the American Bar Association and a Committee of Publishers and Associations.

The information provided herein is stated to be truthful and consistent, in that any liability, in terms of inattention or otherwise, by any usage or abuse of any policies, processes, or directions contained within is the solitary and

backing by the trademark owner. All trademarks and brands within this book are for clarifying purposes only and are owned by the owners themselves, not affiliated with this document.

References

[1] http://ajcn.nutrition.org/content/76/1/266S.short
[2] http://www.ncbi.nlm.nih.gov/pmc/articles/PMC3705319/
[3] http://scienceblog.com/40178/poor-sleep-quality-increases-inflammation-community-study-finds
[4] http://www.ncbi.nlm.nih.gov/pubmed/18296371